MW01490119

LITTLE WONDERS

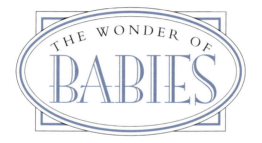

THE WONDER OF
BABIES

Phyllis Hobe

The C.R. Gibson Company
Norwalk, Connecticut 06856

LITTLE WONDERS

The Wonder of Mom
The Wonder of Dad
The Wonder of Friends
The Wonder of Babies
The Wonder of Little Girls
The Wonder of Little Boys

Published by The C.R. Gibson Company,
Norwalk, Connecticut 06856

Printed in the U.S.A.
Designed by Deborah Michel

ISBN 0-8378-7703-2
GB403

Holding a
baby in your arms
makes you feel big,
strong, important,
responsible—and
utterly helpless.

*A baby can turn
your life upside-down
and make it feel right side-up.
A baby can turn your world
around and take it in a
wonderful new direction.*

Each baby

is a separate

miracle.

A baby sees
the world through
your eyes, so you can
rediscover what you
took for granted—
the colors in the sky

before sunrise, the first snowflakes of a winter storm, lacy ice on windows, lights in the night sky, buds opening on a spring morning.

Babies are known
for their patience...
they will wait and wait
and wait until you
finally fall asleep
before they cry.

Babies have
perfect timing...
they will wake from
a sound sleep the
minute you call
a friend.

If you came into
a new world where you
didn't know anyone, and
couldn't speak the language,
and everyone was picking
you up, maybe you'd
cry, too.

When your baby
won't stop crying,
just remember how
thrilled you were when
you heard her voice
for the first time.

A few little hairs
on a baby's head can
create an irresistible
urge to tie a ribbon
around them.

Watch a baby
sleeping at the end
of a day, and you'll
forget how tired
you are.

*A baby's giggle is
a sure cure for stress.*

❧

*A baby's burp is the
ultimate satisfaction.*

A baby's smile can
make you forget whatever
it was you planned to do...
and when you remember,
it didn't matter anyway.

Babies help you
have a sense of humor—
Drooling on the clean
shirt you just put
on is funny...
banging a dent in

the silver rattle your
best friend sent her
is hilarious...
Turning a bowl of
oatmeal upside-down on
her head is a riot!

*W*hen a baby recognizes you, it's better than having your name up in lights.

Giving the first
bath is one of the
bravest things you'll
ever do.

A baby can
introduce you to
the eighth wonder of
the world—
a rocking chair.

You'll learn a
new language with
a new baby.

Did you ever think
that Pat-a-Cake would
turn out to be such
a great game?

Diapering
is a perfectly
logical geometric
exercise.

*D*on't overlook a baby's athletic potential— throwing food clear across the room may indicate a future quarterback...lobbing toys out of a playpen could be the mark of a tennis champ...

crawling at breakneck speed
to push your favorite vase off
the coffee table might mean
a cross country runner...
these are some things to
think about while you're
cleaning up the mess.

There is nothing
as elusive as a baby's mouth
when you're trying to put food in it...
and nothing as accurate as a
baby's aim in blowing food
back at you.

A baby doesn't tie you down...
if you don't mind carrying a bottle,
diapers, a diaper bag, baby powder,
a wash cloth. clean towels, a change
of clothes (yours as well), pacifiers,
assorted rattles and a stroller—
to go out for a loaf of bread.

The first word out
of a baby's mouth isn't
always "Ma-ma" or
"Da-da"—Don't take
it personally if it's
"Bow-wow" or "Kat-kat."

A baby manages
to look exactly like
whichever grandparent
is admiring him.

A baby will charm your mother into thinking she can handle him better than you can. Then she'll be only too happy to baby-sit.

A baby will make
your father forget his
native tongue.

❧❧❧

A baby makes you
take yourself seriously.

*B*abies are very forgiving—
they love to hear you sing,
even if you can't…
and they'll laugh at your jokes,
no matter how many times
you repeat them.

Babies don't need
you to be perfect—
they just need you
to be there.

A baby can
make you wish for
time to yourself...
until finally you get it,
and then you want
your baby back.

Leaving your baby
for the first time is a
lesson in holding
your breath.

Coming home
to a baby who's
been perfectly happy
with someone else is a
relief—or is it?

When babies go visiting, they will not tolerate anyone speaking for more than two minutes— then will demand

silence by howling
at the top of their
lungs. Learn to speak
loudly if you want
to carry on
a conversation.

If your baby cries
when a friend hands
her back to you...
it's because she knows
she doesn't have to
charm you.

Babies like to go to restaurants, but they don't want to eat, they prefer shredding napkins, bouncing rolls, playing with straws, and totally captivating everyone in sight.

A baby
has a temper...
just try removing
the pacifier from her
mouth so you can
take her picture.

Babies come
wrapped in all our
hopes and dreams—
but we have to loosen
the wrappings to give
them space to grow.

As soon as you
figure out a baby's
sleeping, waking and
eating rhythms,
they change.

$\mathcal{W}$hatever works
for your friends'
babies will not work
for yours.

Talking about your
baby in great detail
is perfectly normal...
and a real test of
friendships.

A baby liberates you from trying to do the impossible, such as keeping the house neat and dressing for dinner and always wearing makeup when friends come over.

Every baby is
like every other baby.
Each grows, crawls,
walks and talks at
their own pace.

A baby's first tooth will come in when you're not looking for it.

A baby is an invitation to adventure—seeing his eyes begin to focus... finding out what color they're going to be... feeling his tiny fingers take one of yours captive and never wanting

to be set free... holding your
breath as he stands and tumbles
down into your waiting arms...
and joyful as he gets up again...
cheering as he takes that first
step. The sad thing about
babyhood is that it goes too fast.

Babies aren't prejudiced...
A great aunt's handmade dress
a terry cloth bib and Dad's blue
suit are all the same to them
when it comes to spilling food
all over them.

No one can understand what your baby says— except you.

A baby's steady gaze reminds us that we have a soul and the baby has found it.

*A*ny baby is a
challenge, but your
baby will bring out
the best in you.

A BABY WILL
SEE TO IT THAT YOU
WILL NEVER BE THE SAME—
YOU'LL ALWAYS PUT YOUR
BABY FIRST, BEFORE
ANYONE ELSE, YOU WILL

TAKE LESS FOR YOURSELF
TO GIVE MORE TO YOUR
BABY, YOU'LL TRY TO BE
A BETTER PERSON TO
GIVE YOUR BABY A
BETTER EXAMPLE.

When a baby comes
into your life, you
suddenly understand
your parents.